HISTAMINE INTOLERANCE

FOOD LIST

The Do's and Don'ts

Claudia Adkins

LEGAL DISCLAIMER

This book serves as educational and entertainment material and is not a substitute for professional medical advice or treatment. While the information presented here is sourced from reliable outlets to the best of the Author's knowledge, accuracy cannot be guaranteed. The Author cannot be held responsible for any errors or omissions. It is advisable to consult a medical professional before implementing any remedies or techniques suggested in this book.

By utilizing the information provided, you agree to absolve the Author and Publisher of any liability for damages, expenses, or legal fees arising from the application of the advice contained herein. This disclaimer encompasses any damages or injuries resulting directly or indirectly from the use of the information presented, regardless of the cause of action.

You acknowledge and assume all risks associated with the utilization of the information within this book. It is recommended to consult with a qualified medical practitioner to ensure suitability and safety before engaging in any program outlined herein.

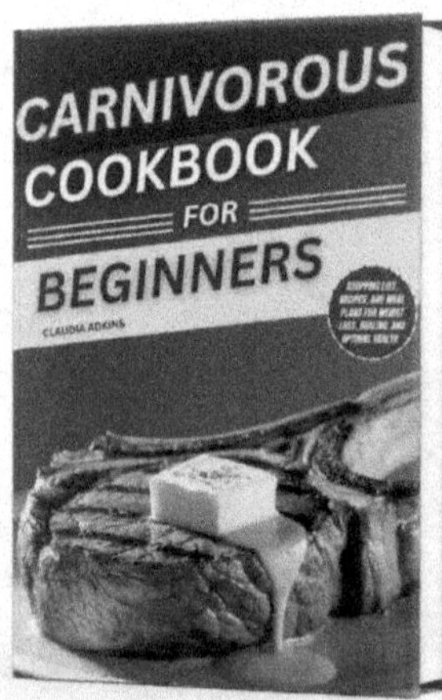

CARNIVOROUS
COOKBOOK
FOR
BEGINNERS
CLAUDIA ADKINS

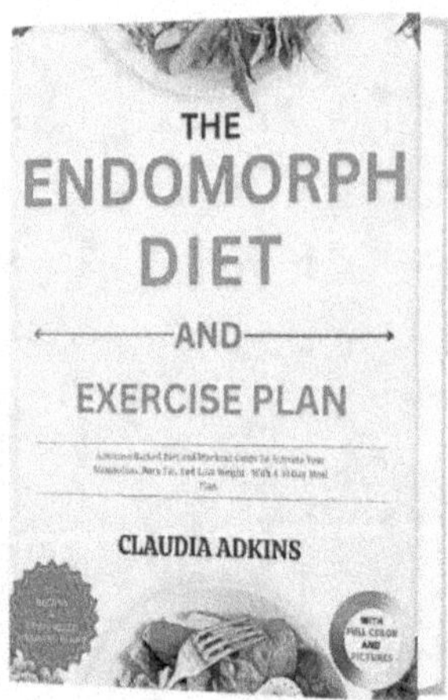

THE
ENDOMORPH
DIET
AND
EXERCISE PLAN
CLAUDIA ADKINS

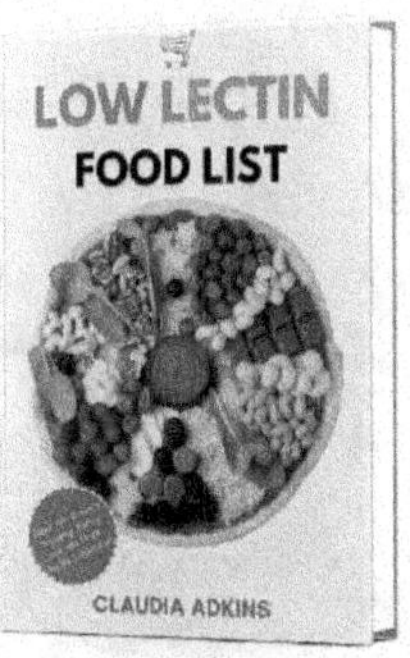

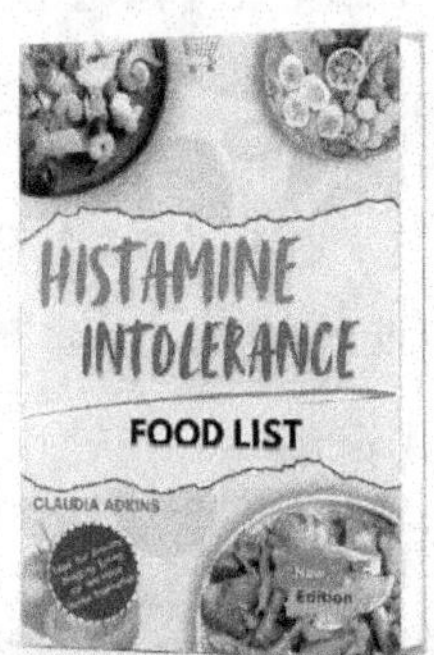

Also available in other languages (German, Spanish, and French

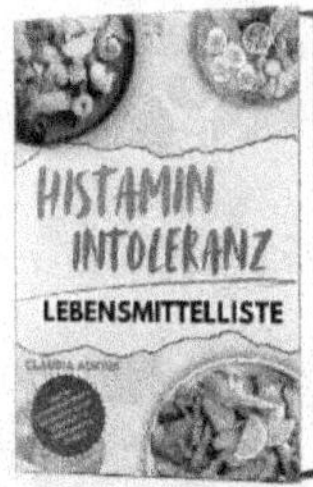

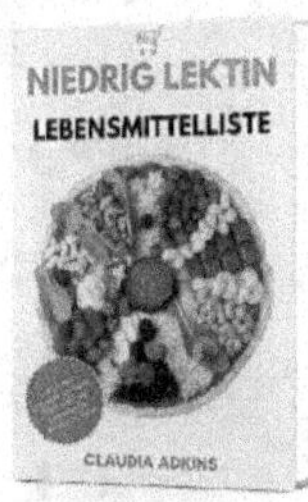

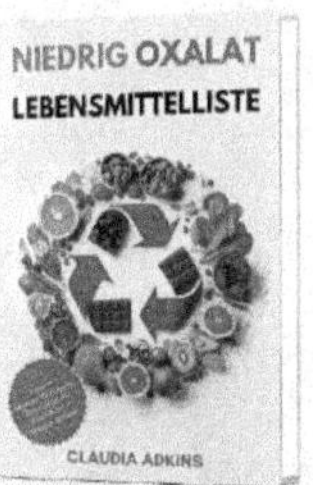

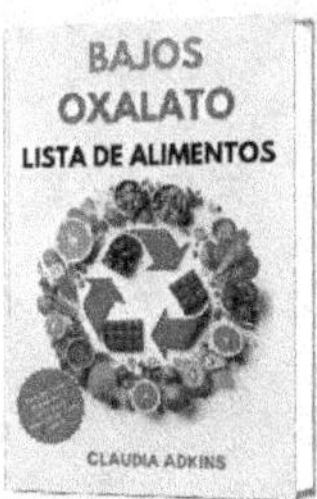

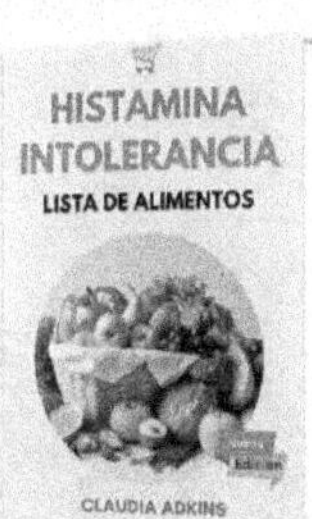

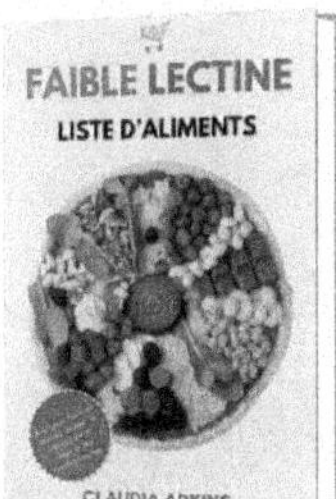

Table of Contents

SOURCES

1. **Histamine Intolerance Awareness Site Food List (Food List)**

Link https://www.histamineintolerance.org.uk/about/the-food-diary/the-food-list/

2. **Alison Vickery Anti-Food List**

Link

https://www.alisonvickery.com/blog/anti-histamine-foods

3. **SFGATE Histamine Reducing Foods**

Link https://healthyeating.sfgate.com/histaminereducing-foods-12197.html

4. **Factvsfitness Master List of Low Histamine Foods**

Link: https://factvsfitness.com/blogs/news/histamine-intolerance-food-list

5. **SIGHI Food List**

Link

https://www.mastzellaktivierung.info/downloads/foodlist/21_FoodList_EN_alphabetic_withCateg.pdf

6. **The Histamine Intolerance Site Food List**

Link

https://histamineintolerance.net/foodlist

7. **MastCell360 Low and High Histamine Food Lists**

Link

https://mastcell360.com/low-histamine-foods-list/

8. **Healing Histamine, Histamine in Food Lists**

Link

https://healinghistamine.com/what-is-histamine/histamine-in-food-lists/

9. **Weekand - Histamine Reducing Foods**

Link

https://www.weekand.com/healthyliving/article/histaminereducing-foods-18013566.php

10. **BBC Good Food**

Link https://www.bbcgoodfood.com

11. **Casa de Sante**

Link https://casadesante.com/blogs/gut-health

12. **Food is Good**

Link

https://foodisgood.com

INTRODUCTION

Welcome to this book! I want to congratulate you on your choice. As someone who also struggles with histamine intolerance, I know how frustrating it can be to find reliable information about what foods to avoid. That's why I put so much effort into creating this guide. I spent a lot of time researching the most trusted dietary information in the world, carefully categorizing foods into low-histamine and high-histamine groups. I even collaborated with talented dieticians and low-histamine cooks to ensure that this book goes beyond just a simple list. This book is not about complicated explanations; it is a practical tool. Although everyone's histamine intolerance may vary, this list provides a strong foundation for your journey. My aim is to simplify your decision-making when it comes to choosing foods. Whether you're shopping for groceries, dining out, or experimenting with new recipes, this book will be your ultimate resource for identifying foods that are likely to have high levels of histamine, trigger its release, or hinder your body's ability to break it down. Let's work together to help you live your best low-histamine life!

This book only contains a list of foods and their histamine levels, but for the sake of those who picked this book for knowledge sake or are having thought about their symptom being caused by histamine intolerance, I appreciate your efforts, and so first before enlisting the foods. I would like to tell you a little about histamine intolerance (HIT).

Histamine Intolerance: The Basics

Okay, so you're wondering if this whole histamine thing might be the culprit behind those annoying headaches or that unpredictable tummy trouble. Let's break it down...

Imagine histamine acting like a little messenger in your body. It does important things, such as helping your immune system fight off intruders. Normally, your body has a team of enzymes (think of them as clean-up crews) called **Diamine oxidase (DAO)** that break down histamine when it's done its job.

But with histamine intolerance, it's like your clean-up crew is either missing members or taking a super long coffee break. Histamine starts piling up, and that's when things get messy. It can cause all sorts of weird symptoms—bloating, headaches, itchy skin, you name it!

So, How Do I Know If It's A HIT?

Unfortunately, there's no quick and easy "histamine intolerance" stamp they can put on your forehead. Here's what you can do:

- **Chat with your doctor:** A good place to start is with a doctor who is knowledgeable about allergies or gut stuff. They'll want to hear all about your symptoms and might suggest some tests.

- **The detective diet:** This means cutting out high-histamine foods for a while, then adding them back in one by one.

It's like playing detective with your body to see what makes it go haywire.

- **The maybe-helpful blood test:** You might get a blood test to check your **Diamine oxidase (DAO) enzyme** levels, but it's not always the answer.

Important stuff to remember:

- **Everyone's a little different.** Some people are super sensitive to even tiny bits of histamine, while others can handle more. It's all about figuring out your limits.

- **It's not an allergy.** This is about your body's cleanup crew, not your immune system going into overdrive, like with a food allergy.

Hopefully, this gives you a clearer picture!

How to Use This Book

Think of this book as your trusty sidekick in your low-histamine journey. Here's how to make it work for you. In the comprehensive list, each food is sorted into simple categories:

- ❖ "Low Histamine" (LH): Generally safer choice and reduces HIT inflammation.
- ❖ "High Histamine" (HH): Best avoided as much as possible
- ❖ **"Debatable levels" (D)**: various research hasn't come to a conclusion or that these foods should be consumed in small portions.
- ❖ "Histamine Liberators" (HL): These don't have much histamine themselves but trigger its release in your body and should also be avoided.
- ❖ **" DAO Blockers " (DB)**: These interfere with your histamine-busting enzyme.

Remember, start slowly and listen to your body. A drastic diet overhaul can be overwhelming! Instead, try gradually reducing high-histamine foods and see how they make you feel. With time, and maybe even with the guidance of your doctor, you might be able to reintroduce some foods to enjoy a more varied diet. Remember, there's no single right way to manage histamine intolerance. Be patient, pay attention to what works for YOU, and use this book as a tool on your journey towards healing and a balanced, healthy life.

Food List

Vegetables and Grains

Algae and algae derivatives

While not technically vegetables, algae derivatives like carrageenan and algin are used as thickeners in various foods, you'll find them in dairy products (like yogurt), non-dairy alternatives (almond milk, vegan cheese), and even some seafood spices. It's wise to research these additives further for informed choices.

❖ **High Histamine (HH)**

Amaranth

Gluten-free grains like amaranth are considered low-histamine-containing foods

❖ **Low Histamine (LH)**

Asparagus

This weight-loss-friendly vegetable has low histamine levels

❖ **Low Histamine (LH)**

Bamboo shoots

This food is said to be low in histamine, but they have been known to trigger HIT allergies in some individuals, especially canned bamboo shoots.

❖ **Debatable levels (D)**

Barley

Barley is considered a low histamine diet, but if you're overly sensitive, I suggest you avoid it.

❖ **Debatable levels (D)**

Barley malt

This grain and food products high in it are considered high in histamine. But its tolerance depends on the individual.

❖ **High Histamine (HH)**

Beetroot

Beetroot is generally considered a low-histamine food, making it suitable for individuals managing histamine intolerance. Its low histamine content allows for inclusion in a low-histamine diet.

❖ Low Histamine (LH)

Bok choi

Bok choy also known as Pak choi is a low-histamine food that can be included in a histamine-restricted diet. Its high nutritional profile offers additional health benefits, making it a valuable addition to various dishes.

❖ Low Histamine (LH)

Broccoli

Broccoli, a member of the cruciferous vegetable family, is renowned for its rich nutrient profile and high anti-inflammatory properties. Broccoli is usually well-tolerated by those sensitive to histamine, as it is a low-histamine food and unlikely to cause histamine release.

❖ Low Histamine (LH)

Brussels sprouts

These cruciferous vegetables are part of the low-histamine diet.

❖ Low Histamine (LH)

Buckwheat

There is a little contradiction about buckwheat being high-histamine food because its peel contains fagopyrine. But buckwheat found in most stores has their peels removed so the grain left is completely low in histamine.

Cabbage

Both green and white cabbage are low-histamine-containing foods.

❖ Low Histamine (LH)

Carrot

In a few studies, it's been reported that while carrots are usually considered low-histamine, they contain small amounts of tyramine, and in some people with histamine intolerance, this might trigger a histamine release.

❖ Low Histamine (LH)
❖ **Debatable levels (D)**

Cassava

Cassava serves as a nutritious and versatile food source, particularly beneficial for individuals seeking low-histamine dietary options. Both cassava and cassava flour are generally considered low in histamine.

- ❖ Low Histamine (LH)

Cassava flour

- ❖ Low Histamine (LH)

Celery

- ❖ Low Histamine (LH)

Cauliflower

Cauliflower is usually regarded as a low-histamine food, which makes it a suitable option for those controlling histamine levels in their diet.

- ❖ Low Histamine (LH)

Watercress

Watercress is typically considered a low-histamine food. Research suggests it also contains compounds, including flavonols and megastigmanes, that may reduce histamine release from mast cells, potentially offering relief from allergy symptoms.

- ❖ Low Histamine (LH)

Cucumber

For those with histamine intolerance, fresh cucumbers are a good choice. However, avoid overripe or pickled cucumbers, as their histamine levels are significantly higher.

❖   Low Histamine (LH)

Endive

Endive is generally classified as a low-histamine food, which makes it suitable for individuals with histamine-related dietary needs.

❖   Low Histamine (LH)

Malt extract

Malt extract is known to raise histamine levels, classifying it as a high-histamine ingredient. Consequently, people with histamine intolerance should generally avoid products containing this ingredient, including some cereals, candies, and baked goods where it functions as a sweetener or flavor enhancer.

❖   High Histamine (HH)

Fennel

For those on a low-histamine diet, fennel, including both its bulb and seeds, is often a suitable option due to its low histamine content.

❖   Low Histamine (LH)

Fennel flower

❖ Low Histamine (LH)

Garlic

Garlic is low in histamine but contains N-acetylcysteine and quercetin which are histamine releasers and DAO blockers.

❖ **DAO Blockers (DB)**
❖ Histamine Liberators (HL)

Pea Sprouts

Pea sprouts have a high concentration of DAO and as such it is very good for breaking down and reducing histamine in the body

❖ Low Histamine (LH)

Moringa

Studies have shown that moringa has antihistamine properties

❖ Low Histamine (LH)

Kohlrabi

Because studies offer no definitive conclusion and individuals report diverse reactions, it's advisable to exclude kohlrabi during elimination diets.

❖ **Debatable levels (D)**

Corn salad

❖ Low Histamine (LH)

Leeks

Leeks have histamine in them but they are not considered as high-histamine foods, so the cause of a reaction highly differs among individuals.

❖ **Debatable levels (D)**

Oats

❖ Low Histamine (LH)

Pak choi

❖ Low Histamine (LH)

Fermented cabbage

Fermented cabbage, widely known as sauerkraut, has a high histamine content that fluctuates depending on the length and temperature of fermentation, along with microbial activity. Therefore, it may be problematic for those managing histamine intolerance.

❖ High Histamine (HH)

Pickled cucumber

❖ High Histamine (HH)

Pickled vegetables

❖ High Histamine (HH)

Potato

❖ Low Histamine (LH)

Quinoa

* ❖ Low Histamine (LH)

Radish

Both red and white have low histamine content.

* ❖ Low Histamine (LH)

Red algae

Red algae is best avoided when following a low-histamine diet because it can contain varying amounts of histamine, is typically rich in iodine, and may act as a histamine liberator, potentially exacerbating histamine-related symptoms.

* ❖ **High Histamine (HH)**
* ❖ Histamine Liberators (HL)

Red cabbage

* ❖ Low Histamine (LH)

Rice

* ❖ Low Histamine (LH)

Black rice

* ❖ Low Histamine (LH)

Spinach

For those with histamine intolerance, spinach is generally considered a food to avoid due to its high histamine content, which increases further as it wilts. However, research suggests that boiling may offer a way to significantly reduce these levels.

❖ **High Histamine (HH)**

Sweet potato

❖ Low Histamine (LH)

Clover

❖ Low Histamine (LH)

Turnip

The suitability of turnip greens for a low-histamine diet is uncertain due to a lack of research on their histamine levels.

❖ **Debatable levels (D)**

Wheat

The histamine content of wheat remains a subject of debate, with certain studies classifying it as low-histamine. However, the relatively high histidine content present in wheat flour can be converted to histamine during processing, particularly through yeast fermentation.

❖ **Debatable levels (D)**

Wheat germ

Wheat germ is identified as a potential histamine liberator, which may elicit histamine release in susceptible individuals.

❖ Histamine Liberators (HL)

Onion (white, red, and yellow)

❖ Low Histamine (LH)

Wild rice

also called lake rice.

- ❖ Low Histamine (LH)

Yam

This rich fibrous root vegetable is considered a low histamine diet.

- ❖ Low Histamine (LH)

Chestnuts

- ❖ Low Histamine (LH)

Sweetcorn

- ❖ Low Histamine (LH)

Horseradish

- ❖ Histamine Liberators (HL)

Olives

Olives are naturally low in histamine when fresh. However, the fermentation or curing processes used for most commercial olives increase their histamine content. Additionally, ripe (black) olives have higher histamine levels compared to unripe (green) olives.

- ❖ **Debatable levels (D)**

Fruits, Nuts, and Seeds

Acerola

Acerola, also known as the **Barbados cherry**, is a small shrub or tree that produces bright red, cherry-like fruits. These little powerhouses are packed with vitamin C, along with other beneficial vitamins and minerals.

❖ Low Histamine (LH)

Almond

Almonds are low in histamine, but they also produce bio-amines that utilize DAO thereby increasing the build-up of histamine. It's advisable to consume almonds in small portions.

❖ **Debatable levels (D)**

Apple

For individuals managing histamine intolerance, apples are generally considered a good choice due to their low histamine content. Furthermore, they are a source of quercetin, a natural antihistamine that may help regulate mast cells and decrease histamine release.

❖ Low Histamine (LH)

Apricot

❖ Low Histamine (LH)

Artichoke

Artichokes, generally low in histamine, are often recommended for those with histamine sensitivities. Their luteolin content, a bioflavonoid, may help prevent histamine release by stabilizing mast cells.

- ❖ Low Histamine (LH)

Eggplant

Eggplant or **aubergine** is known to contain high histamine content, but will not exacerbate the symptoms of HIT in some people.

- ❖ High Histamine (HH)
- ❖ **Debatable levels (D)**

Apple cider vinegar

This vinegar is high in histamine and also causes the body to release histamine.

- ❖ High Histamine (HH)
- ❖ Histamine Liberators (HL)

Chia seed

- ❖ Low Histamine (LH)

Sesame

Sesame seeds are typically low in histamine but contain moderate levels of other biogenic amines that may affect sensitive individuals. Moderation is advised.

- ❖ **Debatable levels (D)**

Avocado

Avocados can be problematic for individuals with histamine intolerance because of their potential histamine content and their ability to release histamine.

- ❖ **High Histamine (HH)**
- ❖ Histamine Liberators (HL)

Banana

Although often considered low-histamine, bananas can act as histamine liberators, and this potential varies with ripeness. Green bananas are less likely to trigger histamine release than ripe bananas, which accumulate histamine as they ripen.

- ❖ Histamine Liberators (HL)
- ❖ **DAO Blockers (DB)**

Bell pepper

- ❖ Low Histamine (LH)

Blackberry

This berry is suitable for a low-histamine diet

- ❖ Low Histamine (LH)

Blackcurrant

- ❖ Low Histamine (LH)

Blueberries

- ❖ Low Histamine (LH)

Boysenberry

❖ Low Histamine (LH)

Brazil nut

Brazil nuts are considered low-histamine foods

❖ Low Histamine (LH)

Dragon fruit

❖ Low Histamine (LH)

Cashew nut

The classification of cashews with respect to histamine content is inconsistent across various sources. Certain experts categorize them as possessing moderate histamine levels, indicating a potential for adverse reactions in highly sensitive individuals. Furthermore, some sources posit that cashews may function as histamine liberators. Individual responses to cashew ingestion exhibit significant variability among individuals with histamine intolerance.

❖ **Debatable levels (D)**

Dates

Dates are low in histamine, but in some individuals, they have been known to cause symptoms because of the sulfite content when it's dried.

❖ Low Histamine (LH)
❖ **Debatable levels (D)**

Flaxseeds

Also known as linseeds.

❖ Low Histamine (LH)

Gooseberry

❖ Low Histamine (LH)

Grapefruit

Despite containing minimal histamine itself, grapefruit is considered a histamine liberator because it can cause the body to release stored histamine.

❖ **High Histamine (HH)**
❖ Histamine Liberators (HL)

Guava

The pulp and skin of guava, particularly in its unripe state, contain histamine as well as proteins capable of eliciting an allergic response, thereby triggering histamine release.

❖ **High Histamine (HH)**

Hazelnuts

Those with histamine intolerance should be mindful of hazelnuts, as they contain histamine-like chemicals and may trigger histamine release, even though they are not inherently high in histamine. Careful monitoring of reactions after consuming small amounts is recommended.

❖ **Debatable levels (D)**

❖ Histamine Liberators (HL)

Kiwi fruit

❖ Histamine Liberators (HL)

Lemon

As with most citrus fruits, lemon fruit or its peel is known to release histamine.

❖ Histamine Liberators (HL)

Lime

❖ Histamine Liberators (HL)

Lingonberry

❖ Low Histamine (LH)

Lychee

❖ Low Histamine (LH)

Watermelon

❖ Histamine Liberators (HL)

Melon

❖ Low Histamine (LH)

Tomatoes

Tomatoes both contain histamine and can induce its release in the body. Tomato-based products contain higher levels of histamine, especially pastes.

❖ Histamine Liberators (HL)

Orange

Orange and its juice both cause the release of histamine.

Pears

Pears are subject to varying classifications regarding their histamine content, with some sources categorizing them as possessing moderate histamine levels. Consequently, caution or avoidance is advised for individuals adhering to a low-histamine dietary regimen.

❖ **Debatable levels (D)**

Persimmon

Pineapple

Despite its low histamine content, pineapple can act as a histamine liberator due to the bromelain it contains, potentially triggering histamine release in some individuals.

Pistachio

Current studies are contradictive on the histamine level in pistachios because its histamine content is low but sometimes triggers the release of histamine in some individuals.

❖ **Debatable levels (D)**

Plum

For those managing histamine intolerance, plums are generally considered a safe choice due to their low histamine content. However, as some sources suggest they may trigger histamine release, it's advisable to eat them in moderation and monitor for any adverse effects.

- ❖ Low Histamine (LH)
- ❖ **Debatable levels (D)**

Pomegranate

- ❖ Low Histamine (LH)

Prune

Most dried fruits are high in histamine.

- ❖ High Histamine (HH)

Psyllium seed husks

- ❖ Low Histamine (LH)

Passion fruit

- ❖ Low Histamine (LH)

Redcurrants

- ❖ Low Histamine (LH)

Rosehip

These little fruits are low in histamine but they are also able to release histamine from the cells.

* ❖ Low Histamine (LH)
* ❖ Histamine Liberators (HL)

Peaches

* ❖ Low Histamine (LH)

Rhubarb

Rhubarb typically exhibits low histamine concentrations; however, certain pre- and post-harvest factors, including stalk maturity and storage conditions, may influence these concentrations. Therefore, it is advisable to consume rhubarb in its fresh state and adhere to appropriate storage protocols to minimize any potential elevation in histamine content.

* ❖ **Debatable levels (D)**

Sharon fruit

* ❖ Low Histamine (LH)

Squash

* ❖ Low Histamine (LH)

Strawberry

* ❖ High Histamine (HH)

Sunflower seed

While sunflower seeds are relatively low in histamine, they contain other biogenic amines that can hinder histamine breakdown and may act as histamine liberators. Improper storage or long shelf life can further increase amine levels, potentially causing symptoms in sensitive individuals.

❖ Histamine Liberators (HL)

Walnut

For individuals with histamine intolerance, walnuts can be problematic as they may trigger histamine release, potentially intensifying symptoms.

❖ Histamine Liberators (HL)

Zucchini

❖ Low Histamine (LH)

Herbs and Spices

Basil

❖ Low Histamine (LH)

Black caraway

Black caraway popularly called **black cumin** spice is very healthy and is considered a low histamine diet.

❖ Low Histamine (LH)

Caraway

❖ Low Histamine (LH)

Cumin

Cumin seeds are low in histamine but these depend on their current situation. When cumin seeds are cool and fresh their histamine levels are low, but if they are poorly stored in warm conditions their histamine content rises and is also known to cause the release of histamine.

- ❖ Low Histamine (LH)

Curry powder

Curry powder typically has low histamine levels. However, variations in spice blends and added ingredients can influence this, so it's important to read labels carefully.

- ❖ Low Histamine (LH)
- ❖ **Debatable levels (D)**

Fenugreek

Research suggests that fenugreek seeds exhibit relatively low histamine concentrations compared to other food sources. While direct investigations into the histamine content of fenugreek leaves are limited, it is plausible to infer a similarly low histamine content in the leaves based on the observed levels in the seeds.

- ❖ **Debatable levels (D)**

Ginger

- ❖ Low Histamine (LH)

Holy Basil

- ❖ Low Histamine (LH)

Black tea

Although black tea itself is typically low in histamine, the presence of other biogenic amines that can slow histamine degradation, combined with the potential for caffeine to inhibit DAO, may be problematic for those with histamine intolerance.

❖ **DAO Blockers (DB)**

Tarragon

❖ Low Histamine (LH)

Nutmeg

Small amounts of nutmeg may be tolerated by some with histamine intolerance due to its moderate histamine content, research indicates that it contains compounds like eugenol and limonene that can act as histamine liberators, potentially causing reactions in sensitive individuals.

❖ **Debatable levels (D)**

Oregano

❖ Low Histamine (LH)

Parsley

❖ Low Histamine (LH)

Paprika (hot)

❖ High Histamine (HH)

Paprika (sweet)

❖ Low Histamine (LH)

Black pepper

  ❖ **High Histamine (HH)**

White pepper

  ❖ **High Histamine (HH)**

Persian cumin

  ❖ Low Histamine (LH)

Galangal

  ❖ Low Histamine (LH)

Turmeric

  ❖ Low Histamine (LH)

Meat extract

  ❖ **High Histamine (HH)**

Coriander

  ❖ Low Histamine (LH)

Rosemary

  ❖ Low Histamine (LH)

Sage

  ❖ Low Histamine (LH)

Star anise seed

In the case of star anise seeds, caution is advised for individuals with histamine intolerance due to the limited available research regarding their histamine content and potential histamine-liberating properties. Discrepancies exist among sources, with some suggesting low histamine concentrations and others cautioning against potential histamine release.

❖ **Debatable levels (D)**

Cinnamon

❖ High Histamine (HH)

Thyme

❖ Low Histamine (LH)

Vanilla

Vanilla is low in histamine but can cause reactions in some people so it should be consumed in low quantities. This applies to all vanilla products (vanilla sugar, vanilla powder, vanilla extract)

❖ **Debatable levels (D)**

Proteins (Meat, Poultry, Fish, and Dairy)

Egg whites

Once thought to trigger histamine release, research suggests they're likely low-histamine.

❖ **Debatable levels (D)**

Egg yolk

Egg yolk does contain histamine but in very low amounts.

- ❖ Low Histamine (LH)

Non-organic meat

These are known to have high histamine levels especially if they have overstayed unrefrigerated for a long time.

- ❖ High Histamine (HH)

Anchovies

Yes, anchovies are known for their high histamine content but keep in mind that this can fluctuate depending on their freshness and how they are processed.

- ❖ High Histamine (HH)

Smoked meat

Smoked meat like salami and sausages are known to have high histamine

- ❖ High Histamine (HH)

Beef

When fresh, frozen, or cooled beef is considered a low-histamine food. However aged meat is considered a high-histamine food

- ❖ **Debatable levels (D)**

Cheese

Aged cheese, such as mold cheese, blue cheese, and cheddar are the most common products responsible for HIT allergies.

❖ High Histamine (HH)

Chicken

Fresh or frozen chicken is a good low-histamine choice. Avoid older or improperly stored chicken, as it becomes high in histamine due to spoilage.

❖ Low Histamine (LH)

Bouillon

Store-bought beef bouillon and broth are often high in histamine due to ingredients like yeast extract, glutamate, and histamine-containing spices.

❖ High Histamine (HH)

Butterkäse

❖ Low Histamine (LH)

Buttermilk

Due to its fermented nature, it's considered a high histamine-containing food.

❖ High Histamine (HH)

Cream

When there are no additives, cream is considered a low-histamine food.

❖ Low Histamine (LH)

Sourcream

Sour cream does contain histamine; however, its concentrations are typically lower than those found in aged cheeses and other dairy products with elevated histamine levels. Notably, histamine formation occurs rapidly following exposure to air after opening. It is important to acknowledge that dietary triggers are subject to individual variability.

❖ **Debatable levels (D)**

Dried meat

❖ High Histamine (HH)

Minced meat (fresh)

The histamine content of minced meat is contingent upon its time since production. When consumed immediately after mincing, histamine concentrations are low; however, minced meat available for **open sale or in pre-packaged** form exhibits **elevated histamine** concentrations.

❖ Low Histamine (LH)

Duck

Fresh or frozen duck is a good low-histamine choice. Avoid older or improperly stored duck, as it becomes high in histamine due to spoilage.

❖ Low Histamine (LH)

Eggs (whole eggs)

❖ High Histamine (HH)

Yogurt

The histamine level of yogurt varies as it depends on the kind of bacteria (probiotics) used during production.

❖ **Debatable levels (D)**

Sheep's milk

This is considered a low-histamine food as long as it's refrigerated or fresh.

❖ Low Histamine (LH)

Pasteurized milk

❖ Low Histamine (LH)

Feta cheese

❖ High Histamine (HH)

Cottage cheese

❖ Low Histamine (LH)

Fish

Fish is low in histamine when fresh (within an hour) or frozen (within an hour).

❖   Low Histamine (LH)

Fish (stored or iced)

Fish in store racks or ice have their histamine content increased.

❖   High Histamine (HH)

Smoked fish

❖   High Histamine (HH)

Fontina cheese

❖   High Histamine (HH)

Hard cheese

❖   High Histamine (HH)

Raclette cheese

❖   High Histamine (HH)

Geheimrats cheese

Also known as Geheimratskaese.

❖   Low Histamine (LH)

Game (meat)

While fresh game meats (e.g., venison, bison, elk, rabbit, boar, and ostrich) typically have low histamine levels due to their wild nature and natural diets, processing and storage methods can significantly affect their histamine content. Aging, curing, or improper storage can elevate histamine, potentially causing issues for those with histamine intolerance.

And, even fresh game meat has its histamine levels higher than that farmed meat

- ❖ **Debatable levels (D)**

Gouda cheese

As with most fermented foods, aged gouda cheese has high histamine levels.

- ❖ High Histamine (HH)

Lamb

Freshly cooked lamb is a preferable low-histamine meat.

- ❖ Low Histamine (LH)

Langouste

Lobsters are low in histamine when freshly caught or immediately frozen, but most times store bought lobsters contain high amounts of histamine

- ❖ High Histamine (HH)

Mozzarella

- ❖ Low Histamine (LH)

Mascarpone

- ❖ Low Histamine (LH)

Milk powder

❖ **Debatable levels (D)**

Ostrich

As wild games, they have low histamine levels, provided they are still fresh.

❖ Low Histamine (LH)

Oyster

❖ High Histamine (HH)

Canned tuna

❖ High Histamine (HH)

Canned meat

❖ High Histamine (HH)

Pork

Pork meat is low in histamine only if it's fresh or frozen immediately.

❖ Low Histamine (LH)

Processed cheese

❖ High Histamine (HH)

Prawn

❖ Histamine Liberators (HL)

Quail eggs

❖ Low Histamine (LH)

Quail

This bird meat is low in histamine only if it's fresh or frozen immediately.

- ❖ Low Histamine (LH)

Rabbit

Low in histamine only if it's fresh or frozen immediately.

- ❖ Low Histamine (LH)

Raw milk

- ❖ Low Histamine (LH)

Rice milk

Rice is a low histamine food but in rice milk other substances may influence the histamine level of the milk.

- ❖ **Debatable levels (D)**

Ricotta cheese

An unaged ricotta cheese has low histamine content.

- ❖ Low Histamine (LH)

Roquefort cheese

Because of the extensive aging and fermentation involved in its production, Roquefort cheese is classified as high-histamine.

- ❖ High Histamine (HH)

Salami

❖ **High Histamine (HH)**

Salmon

Only when fresh or immediately frozen within an hour can salmon be eaten as a low-histamine food.

❖ **High Histamine (HH)**

Sausage

The fermentation and aging processes involved in making processed sausages like salami and pepperoni result in increased histamine content.

❖ **High Histamine (HH)**

Shellfish

❖ **High Histamine (HH)**

Clams

❖ **High Histamine (HH)**

Mussels

❖ **High Histamine (HH)**

Turkey

For a low-histamine choice, opt for fresh turkey or make sure it's been frozen within an hour of slaughter.

❖ **Low Histamine (LH)**

Veal

Low in histamine only if it's fresh or frozen immediately.

❖ Low Histamine (LH)

Whey

❖ Low Histamine (LH)

Oils

Black caraway oil

This oil as well as its seed counterpart is considered a low histamine diet.

❖ Low Histamine (LH)

Butter

Butter is low in histamine. Although some people have different triggers.

❖ Low Histamine (LH)

Fennel flower oil

❖ Low Histamine (LH)

Lard

❖ Low Histamine (LH)

Nutmeg flower oil

❖ Low Histamine (LH)

Palm kernel oil

❖ Low Histamine (LH)

Pumpkin seed oil

❖ Low Histamine (LH)

Canola oil

Also known as rapeseed oil.

❖ Low Histamine (LH)

Coriander oil

❖ Low Histamine (LH)

Olive oil

❖ Low Histamine (LH)

Sunflower oil

Sunflower oil is considered as a high-histamine food when used for a long period.

❖ **Debatable levels (D)**

Walnut oil

Walnuts themselves are not inherently high in histamine; however, the presence of other biogenic amines and their potential to induce histamine release may provoke reactions in sensitive individuals.

❖ Histamine Liberators (HL)

Drinks, Smoothies, and Sweeteners

Agave syrup

While there are contradictions in sweeteners like agave syrup containing high histamine, it's been discovered that natural agave syrup with no additives contains very low histamine.

- ❖ Low Histamine (LH)

Maple syrup

Maple syrup is another sweetener considered safe

- ❖ Low Histamine (LH)

Stevia

- ❖ Low Histamine (LH)

Alcohol and Alcoholic beverages

Alcoholic drinks such as **beer, wine, and cider** have been reported to have higher levels of histamine. But drinks like **plain vodka, gin, and white rum** are all low in histamine, still, take these in moderation or best, cut it off completely.

- ❖ DAO Blockers (DB)
- ❖ High Histamine (HH)

Artificial sweeteners

Consuming too many artificial sweeteners can potentially lead to increased inflammation, which is known to promote histamine release.

- ❖ **High Histamine (HH)**
- ❖ Histamine Liberators (HL)

Brandy

The distillation process employed in the production of spirits such as brandy typically results in a reduction of histamine concentrations compared to non-distilled alcoholic beverages like wine or beer. Nonetheless, brandy may still contain residual histamine and functions as a histamine liberator, inducing the release of endogenous histamine. Additionally, alcohol exerts an inhibitory effect on diamine oxidase (DAO).

- ❖ **DAO Blockers (DB)**
- ❖ **High Histamine (HH)**
- ❖ Histamine Liberators (HL)

Coca Cola

Coca-Cola itself is histamine-free, but ingredients like caffeine and certain preservatives (e.g., sodium benzoate) may trigger histamine release in sensitive individuals. Moderation is advised.

- ❖ **Debatable levels (D)**

Chamomile tea

- ❖ Low Histamine (LH)

Champagne

❖ **High Histamine (HH)**

Dextrose

❖ Low Histamine (LH)

Energy drinks

Although energy drinks are not usually high in histamine, they can affect histamine levels through two main mechanisms: caffeine can increase cortisol, which in turn elevates histamine, and ingredients such as guarana and mate has been identified as DAO inhibitors. Alternatively, you can get a gentle energy lift from low histamine herbal varieties like chamomile or rooibos.

❖ High Histamine (HH)

❖ **DAO Blockers (DB)**

Espresso

While espresso is recognized for its rich and flavorful characteristics, its histamine concentration and the physiological effects of caffeine may pose concerns for individuals with histamine intolerance.

❖ High Histamine (HH)

❖ **DAO Blockers (DB)**

Fructose

❖ Low Histamine (LH)

Honey

❖   Low Histamine (LH)

Chocolate

Chocolate doesn't have a lot of histamine, but it can trigger your body to release its own stored histamine. Additionally, it contains compounds that can make it harder for your body to break down histamine.

❖   **DAO Blockers (DB)**

❖   Histamine Liberators (HL)

Lactose

❖   Low Histamine (LH)

Lemonade

❖   Histamine Liberators (HL)

Peppermint tea

❖   Low Histamine (LH)

Rooibos tea

❖   Low Histamine (LH)

Green tea

Green tea generally exhibits low histamine concentrations due to the absence of fermentation in its production. Moreover, it contains catechins, notably epigallocatechin gallate (EGCG), which have demonstrated the capacity to inhibit histamine release from mast cells. This suggests a potential mitigating effect on histamine-related symptoms. However, individual responses to green tea consumption can vary considerably. Some individuals with histamine intolerance may still experience adverse reactions, potentially attributable to the caffeine content, which, in higher concentrations, can inhibit the activity of diamine oxidase (DAO). Consequently, it is advisable to initiate consumption with a small quantity and seek guidance from a healthcare professional.

- ❖ **Debatable levels (D)**

Lime blossom tea

- ❖ Low Histamine (LH)

Rum

- ❖ High Histamine (HH)

Sage tea

- ❖ Low Histamine (LH)

Schnapps

- ❖ High Histamine (HH)

Soda

Due to unknown levels of histamine in added sweeteners in sodas, it can be considered to contain histamine.

- ❖ **Debatable levels (D)**
- ❖ High Histamine (HH)

Soft drinks

Despite their typically low histamine content, soft drinks can pose challenges for those with histamine intolerance due to two main factors: the caffeine they often contain, which can inhibit DAO, and the presence of artificial additives that may trigger histamine release or hinder its breakdown. Therefore, **moderation** and choosing low-histamine alternatives are advisable.

❖ **Debatable levels (D)**

Soy milk

The histamine content of soy milk is influenced by several factors, including processing methods and storage conditions. Fermentation significantly increases histamine levels, as seen in products like tempeh and miso. Even unfermented soy milk, typically low to moderate in histamine, may still cause reactions in highly sensitive individuals.

❖ High Histamine (HH)

Sucrose

❖ Low Histamine (LH)

Spirits

❖ High Histamine (HH)

Verbena herbal tea

❖ Low Histamine (LH)

Wine (histamine-free)

Even histamine-free wines should be taking with caution as individual responses varies.

❖ **Debatable levels (D)**

Wine (Schilcher wein)

❖ **High Histamine (HH)**

Legumes

Beans

❖ **High Histamine (HH)**
❖ Histamine Liberators (HL)

Peanuts.

❖ **High Histamine (HH)**
❖ Histamine Liberators (HL)

Soybeans.

❖ **High Histamine (HH)**
❖ Histamine Liberators (HL)

Peas

❖ **High Histamine (HH)**
❖ Histamine Liberators (HL)

Kidney beans.

❖ **High Histamine (HH)**

❖ Histamine Liberators (HL)

Chickpeas.

- ❖ **High Histamine (HH)**
- ❖ Histamine Liberators (HL)

Green beans

Green beans typically exhibit low histamine concentrations. However, certain sources suggest they may possess histamine-liberating properties, potentially inducing the release of endogenous histamine and eliciting symptoms in susceptible individuals. Nonetheless, individual responses vary considerably, and many individuals with histamine intolerance tolerate green beans without experiencing adverse reactions.

- ❖ **Debatable levels (D)**
- ❖ Histamine Liberators (HL)

Borlotti beans

- ❖ **High Histamine (HH)**
- ❖ Histamine Liberators (HL)

Fava bean

Also known as broad bean

- ❖ **High Histamine (HH)**

Beansprout

This is one of the few legumes that are considered low-histamine food because it's a good source of DAO

Lentils

Despite their low histamine content, lentils contain other biogenic amines that can interfere with histamine breakdown by competing for the DAO enzyme. This interference could lead to elevated histamine levels in sensitive individuals. Additionally, some sources suggest lentils may act as histamine liberators. Individual reactions vary.

❖ Low Histamine (LH)
❖ **Debatable levels (D)**

Pulses

❖ High Histamine (HH)

Extras

Bread

Bread and gluten foods have high amounts of histamine due to their fermentation process. However, some breads, like soda bread, can be low in histamine.

❖ High Histamine (HH)

Penny bun

These fungi are low in histamine but in some individuals, they can trigger the release of histamine.

❖ Low Histamine (LH)

❖ Histamine Liberators (HL)

Distilled white vinegar

❖ Low Histamine (LH)

Hemp seeds

❖ Low Histamine (LH)

Peppermints

❖ Low Histamine (LH)

Eggnog

Eggnog can pose problems for those with histamine intolerance through several mechanisms. Dairy and raw egg whites may contain histamine and act as liberators. Nutmeg and cinnamon can raise histamine levels in sensitive individuals. Furthermore, alcohol, frequently an ingredient in eggnog, can inhibit DAO activity.

❖ High Histamine (HH)

Corn Pasta

❖ Low Histamine (LH)

Gelatin

❖ Histamine Liberators (HL)

Porcino mushroom

Fresh porcino mushrooms are considered edible for a low-histamine diet. But these may still cause HIT in some individuals due to the presence of histamine-like amines.

❖ **Debatable levels (D)**

Red wine vinegar

❖ **High Histamine (HH)**

Morel

❖ **High Histamine (HH)**

Mushrooms

Different types. Although mushrooms are generally low in histamine, they contain other amines that can produce similar effects to histamine intolerance. Therefore, it's best to consume them in moderation or avoid them altogether.

❖ **Debatable levels (D)**

Rice crispies

❖ **Low Histamine (LH)**

Rice noodle

❖ **Low Histamine (LH)**

Additives with hydrolyzed plant protein

❖ **Low Histamine (LH)**
❖ **Histamine Liberators (HL)**

Seafood

❖ High Histamine (HH)

Seaweed

❖ High Histamine (HH)

Soy sauce

❖ High Histamine (HH)

Soy protein powder

❖ High Histamine (HH)

Starch

❖ Low Histamine (LH)

Tiger nut

❖ Low Histamine (LH)

Balsamic vinegar

❖ High Histamine (HH)

Yeast

While yeast itself is not a significant source of histamine, its role in food processing, particularly fermentation and leavening, can lead to histamine production. Yeast extract is a notable exception, containing high levels of biogenic amines, including histamine, and potentially inhibiting DAO. The histamine content of nutritional yeast is inconsistent across sources. Baker's and brewer's yeast, used in baking and brewing, don't inherently contain much histamine but contribute to its formation during fermentation. Therefore, those with histamine intolerance should exercise caution with yeast-containing foods.

❖ **Debatable levels (D)**

Yeast extract
❖ High Histamine (HH)

Food Additives

Azorubine (food red 3)
❖ High Histamine (HH)

Carmine
❖ High Histamine (HH)

Curcumin, E100
❖ Low Histamine (LH)

Erythrosine, E127
❖ High Histamine (HH)

Indigo carmine
❖ **Debatable levels (D)**

Plain caramel

Plain caramel as well as E150a (caustic caramel) are part of low histamine food additives.

❖ Low Histamine (LH)

Quinoline yellow

Food Yellow 13, E104

❖ **High Histamine (HH)**

❖ Histamine Liberators (HL)

Orange yellow S, E110

❖ **High Histamine (HH)**

Tartrazine, E102

❖ **High Histamine (HH)**

Benzoates (E210-213)

❖ **High Histamine (HH)**

Salicylic acid

❖ **High Histamine (HH)**

Sodium nitrite, E250

❖ Low Histamine (LH)

Sulfites

❖ **High Histamine (HH)**

Calcium diglutamate, E623

  ❖ **High Histamine (HH)**

Glutamates (E620-625)

  ❖ **High Histamine (HH)**

Monosodium glutamate (MSG)

  ❖ **High Histamine (HH)**

Monoammonium glutamate

  ❖ **High Histamine (HH)**

Potassium glutamate

  ❖ **High Histamine (HH)**

Pectin

  ❖ **Low Histamine (LH)**

Guar gum

  ❖ **High Histamine (HH)**

Cream of tartar

  ❖ **Low Histamine (LH)**

Processed seaweed (E407, E407a)

  ❖ **High Histamine (HH)**

Ascorbic acid

Although low in histamine, vitamin E300 or ascorbic acid blocks DAO

- ❖ Low Histamine (LH)
- ❖ **DAO Blockers (DB)**

Citric acid, E330

- ❖ Low Histamine (LH)

Quinine

- ❖ **High Histamine (HH)**

Folic acid

- ❖ **High Histamine (HH)**
- ❖ Histamine Liberators (HL)

Iodine

- ❖ **High Histamine (HH)**
- ❖ Histamine Liberators (HL)

Potassium iodide

- ❖ **High Histamine (HH)**
- ❖ Histamine Liberators (HL)

Theobromine

- ❖ **DAO Blockers (DB)**

Mustard

- ❖ **High Histamine (HH)**
- ❖ Histamine Liberators (HL)

Tofu

- ❖ **High Histamine (HH)**
- ❖ Histamine Liberators (HL)

____

Notes

____

<u>Trigger foods</u>

<u>**Preferred recipes**</u>

<u>**Restaurant recommendations**</u>

Trigger foods

<u>Preferred recipes</u>

<u>**Restaurant recommendations**</u>

Appendix

Beans	69
Beansprout	70
Beef	52
Beetroot	29
Bell pepper	40
Benzoates (E210-213	76
Black caraway	47
Black caraway oil	61
Black pepper	50
Black rice	35
Black tea	49
Blackberry	40
Blackcurrant	40
Blueberries	40
Bok choi	29
Borlotti beans	70
Bouillon	53
Boysenberry	41
Brandy	64
Brazil nut	41
Bread	71
Broccoli	29
Brussels sprouts	30
Buckwheat	30
Butter	61
Butterkäse	53
Buttermilk	53
Cabbage	30

Calcium diglutamate, E623	77
Canned meat	58
Canned tuna	58
Canola oil	62
Caraway	47
Carmine	75
Carrot	30
Cashew nut	41
Cassava	31
Cassava flour	31
Cauliflower	31
Celery	31
Chamomile tea	64
Champagne	65
Cheese	53
Chestnuts	37
Chia seed	39
Chicken	53
Chickpeas.	70
Chocolate	66
Cinnamon	51
Citric acid, E330	78
Clams	60
Clover	36
Coca Cola	64
Coriander	50
Coriander oil	62
Corn Pasta	72

Corn salad	33
Cottage cheese	55
Cream	54
Cream of tartar	77
Cucumber	32
Cumin	48
Curcumin, E100	75
Curry powder	48
Dates	41
Dextrose	65
Distilled white vinegar	72
Dragon fruit	41
Dried meat	54
Duck	55
Egg whites	51
Egg yolk	52
Eggnog	72
Eggplant	39
Eggs (whole eggs)	55
Endive	32
Energy drinks	65
Erythrosine, E127	75
Espresso	65
Fava bean	70
Fennel	32
Fennel flower	33
Fennel flower oil	61
Fenugreek	48

Fermented cabbage	34
Feta cheese	55
Fish	56
Fish (stored or iced)	56
Flaxseeds	42
Folic acid	78
Fontina cheese	56
Fructose	65
Galangal	50
Game (meat)	56
Garlic	33
Geheimrats cheese	56
Gelatin	72
Ginger	48
Glutamates (E620-625)	77
Gooseberry	42
Gouda cheese	57
Grapefruit	42
Green beans	70
Green tea	66
Guar gum	77
Guava	42
Hard cheese	56
Hazelnuts	42
Hemp seeds	72
Holy Basil	48
Honey	66
Horseradish	37

Indigo carmine	75
Iodine	78
Kidney beans.	69
Kiwi fruit	43
Kohlrabi	33
Lactose	66
Lamb	57
Langouste	57
Lard	61
Leeks	34
Lemon	43
Lemonade	66
Lentils	71
Lime	43
Lime blossom tea	67
Lingonberry	43
Lychee	43
Malt extract	32
Maple syrup	63
Mascarpone	57
Meat extract	50
Melon	43
Milk powder	58
Minced meat (fresh)	54
Monoammonium glutamate	77
Monosodium glutamate (MSG)	77
Morel	73
Moringa	33

Mozzarella	57
Mushrooms	73
Mussels	60
Mustard	78
Non-organic meat	52
Nutmeg	49
Nutmeg flower oil	61
Oats	34
Olive oil	62
Olives	37
Onion (white, red, and yellow)	36
Orange	44
Orange yellow S, E110	76
Oregano	49
Ostrich	58
Oyster	58
Pak choi	34
Palm kernel oil	62
Paprika (hot)	49
Paprika (sweet)	49
Parsley	49
Passion fruit	45
Pasteurized milk	55
Pea Sprouts	33
Peaches	46
Peanuts.	69
Pears	44
Peas	69

Pectin	77
Penny bun	71
Peppermint tea	66
Peppermints	72
Persian cumin	50
Persimmon	44
Pickled cucumber	34
Pickled vegetables	34
Pineapple	44
Pistachio	44
Plain caramel	76
Plum	45
Pomegranate	45
Porcino mushroom	73
Pork	58
Potassium glutamate	77
Potassium iodide	78
Potato	34
Prawn	58
Processed cheese	58
Processed seaweed (E407, E407a)	77
Prune	45
Psyllium seed husks	45
Pulses	71
Pumpkin seed oil	62
Quail	59
Quail eggs	58

Quinine	78
Quinoa	35
Quinoline yellow	76
Rabbit	59
Raclette cheese	56
Radish	35
Raw milk	59
Red algae	35
Red cabbage	35
Red wine vinegar	73
Redcurrants	45
Rhubarb	46
Rice	35
Rice crispies	73
Rice milk	59
Rice noodle	73
Ricotta cheese	59
Rooibos tea	66
Roquefort cheese	59
Rosehip	45
Rosemary	50
Rum	67
Sage	50
Sage tea	67
Salami	60
Salicylic acid	76
Salmon	60
Sausage	60

Schnapps	67
Seafood	74
Seaweed	74
Sesame	39
Sharon fruit	46
Sheep's milk	55
Shellfish	60
Smoked fish	56
Smoked meat	52
Soda	67
Sodium nitrite, E250	76
Soft drinks	68
Sourcream	54
Soy milk	68
Soy protein powder	74
Soy sauce	74
Soybeans.	69
Spinach	35
Spirits	68
Squash	46
Star anise seed	50
Starch	74
Stevia	63
Strawberry	46
Sucrose	68
Sulfites	76
Sunflower oil	62
Sunflower seed	46

Sweet potato	36
Sweetcorn	37
Tarragon	49
Tartrazine, E102	76
Theobromine	78
Thyme	51
Tiger nut	74
Tofu	78
Tomatoes	43
Turkey	60
Turmeric	50
Turnip	36
Vanilla	51
Veal	61
Verbena herbal tea	68
Walnut	47
Walnut oil	62
Watercress	31
Watermelon	43
Wheat	36
Wheat germ	36
Whey	61
White pepper	50
Wild rice	37
Wine (histamine-free)	69
Wine (Schilcher wein)	69
Yam	37
Yeast	74

Yeast extract	75
Yogurt	55
Zucchini	47